Homemade Oral Care

60 Natural Recipes of Toothpaste and Lip Balms

Table of Contents

Introduction 5

Chapter 1. Collection of Homemade Toothpastes 6

Chapter 2. Collection of Homemade Mouthwash Recipes 19

Bonus DIY Anti-Cold Lip Balms & Kids Fun Lip Balms Recipe Collection 33

Conclusion 50

Introduction

I would first like to thank and congratulate you for downloading my book *"Homemade Oral Care: 40 Natural Herbal Recipes to Take Care of Your Teeth and Oral Cavity!"* You will enjoy being able to make your own oral care products from natural ingredients that you know are not filled with harmful chemicals and other man-made additives. Making your own oral care products is going to help you to be much more self-sufficient.

Having this know-how will certainly come in very handy when you could find yourself with limited resources. You could find that products might not be available to you as they once were due to some kind of emergency situation you could find yourself in.

Of course I hope that you will never find yourself in this type of situation, but it is a good idea to help prepare yourself for situations where you may need to become more resourceful with what items you have at hand. Doing this will help you to become less reliant on store bought products and more things such as oral care products that are homemade using natural herbal ingredients.

To get you started I have collected a wonderful assortment of oral care recipes for you to try. I have also included some wonderful bonus recipes for anti-cold lip balms and kid's lip balm recipes that your child will surely love! This is a project that you could both do together that is easy and simple. It can offer you some fun quality time connecting with your child!

Chapter 1. Collection of Homemade Toothpastes

1. Coconut Oil & Clay Toothpaste

Ingredients:

- 1/3 of a cup of boiling water

- 2 tablespoons of coconut oil

- 1/4 of a teaspoon of fine sea salt

- 2 teaspoons of peppermint extract

- 3 teaspoons of xylitol

- 1/4 of a cup of Redmond Clay

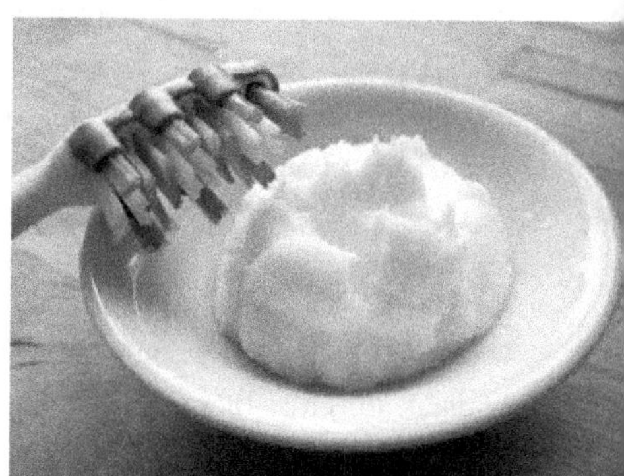

Directions:

Place the water into a pan and place it over medium heat and bring it to a boil. Mix clay and sea salt in a bowl. Add the water into the bowl after it is boiled. Mix using a hand mixer. Add your remaining ingredients into bowl and mix well. Keep toothpaste mix in an airtight container.

2. Coconut Oil Toothpaste

Ingredients:

- 1 packet of Stevia

- 2 teaspoons of vegetable glycerin

- 25 drops of peppermint essential oil

- 3 tablespoons of baking soda

- 3 tablespoons of coconut oil

Directions:

Mix together in a bowl your baking soda and coconut oil. Use a fork to mash to make sure that the mix is thoroughly blended. Add in the remaining ingredients and mash until a paste has formed. Transfer the paste into small glass jar to store with airtight lid.

3. Peppermint & Cinnamon Toothpaste

Ingredients:

- 20 drops of peppermint essential oil
- 20 drops of cinnamon essential oil
- 4 tablespoons of raw honey
- 2 teaspoons of fine sea salt
- 1 tablespoon of magnesium, powdered
- 2 tablespoons of coral calcium
- 1 tablespoon of coconut oil
- one-half cup of olive oil

Directions:

Place glass jar into a bowl of warm water. Add the honey and oils into the jar. Once the coconut oil has melted, add in your minerals, oils and sea salt. Mix well with a hand blender. Keep in a dark glass jar with a soap pump. Shake jar well before each use.

4. Geranium Rose Toothpaste

Ingredients:

- 20 drops of rose essential oils

- 20 drops of geranium essential oils

- 3 tablespoons of raw honey

- 4 teaspoons of tincture of vanilla

- 3 ounces of orris root, powdered

- 1/2 an ounce of powdered chalk

Directions:

Place all of your ingredients into a bowl and mix until a paste is formed. Transfer this paste to an airtight container. You can apply paste using a Popsicle stick, when adding paste to toothbrush.

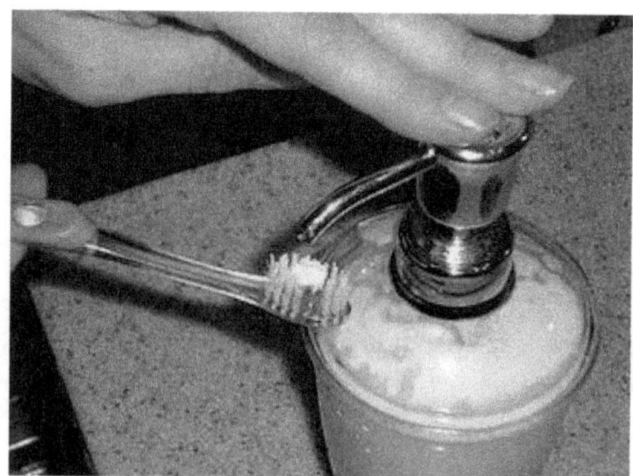

5. *Rose Geranium & Vanilla Toothpaste*

Ingredients:

- 15 drops of rose geranium essential oils

- 4 teaspoons of tincture of vanilla

- 4 tablespoons of raw honey

- 3 ounces of orris root, powdered

- 1/2 ounce of powdered chalk

Directions:

Mix your ingredients in a large bowl until a paste has formed. Store the paste in an airtight container. Use a Popsicle stick to apply paste to your toothbrush.

6. *Clove Coconut-Base Toothpaste*

Ingredients:

- 10 drops of clove pure essential oil

- 2 tablespoons of melted coconut oil

- 1/4 of a teaspoon of hydrogen peroxide

- 7 teaspoons of baking soda

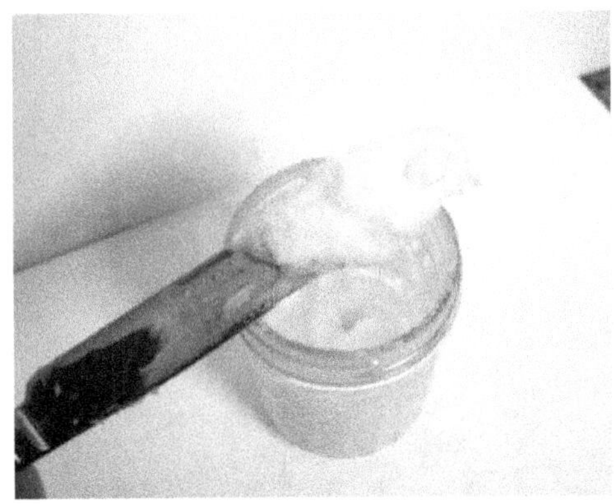

Directions:

Add your ingredients into a mixing bowl, mix well until a paste has formed. Store in an opaque container.

7. Vegan Citrus Toothpaste

Ingredients:

- 6 drops of citrus pure essential oil

- 8 tablespoons of water

- 1/2 a teaspoon of guar gum

- 4 tablespoons of baking soda

- 3 teaspoons of vegetable glycerin

Directions:

Mix the baking soda, vegetable glycerin, guar gum and water in a pot over low heat for five minutes. This mixture should have the consistency of a paste. Remove pot from heat and allow it to cool. Add in the oil, stirring it into the mix. Transfer mix into dark glass jar with airtight lid.

8. Basic Peppermint Toothpaste

Ingredients:

- 4 teaspoons of water

- 4 drops of peppermint essential oil

- 1/2 a teaspoon of fine sea salt

- 1 teaspoon of baking soda

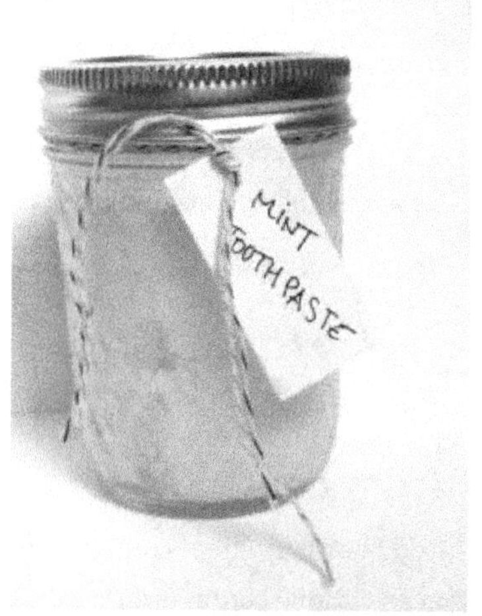

Directions:

In a small mixing bowl blend your ingredients. Mix them until a paste has formed. Transfer the paste to small opaque jar with airtight lid.

9. Cinnamon Toothpaste

Ingredients:

- 5 drops of cinnamon pure essential oil
- 2 tablespoons of hot water
- 1/2 a teaspoon of fine sea salt
- 5 tablespoons of Bentonite clay

Directions:

Mix your ingredients in a mixing bowl, blending until a paste forms. Transfer your paste into a dark glass jar with airtight lid.

10. Spearmint Toothpaste

Ingredients:

- 5 drops of water
- 4 drops of spearmint essential oil
- 1/2 teaspoon of fine sea salt
- 1 teaspoon of baking soda

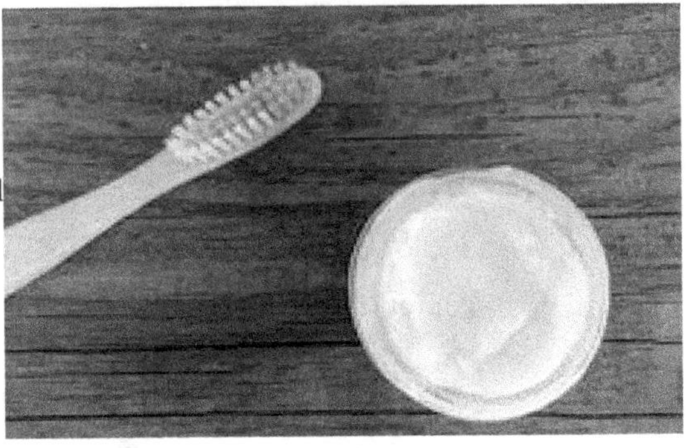

Directions:

Mix all of your toothpaste ingredients until a paste has formed in a bowl. Transfer into small airtight container with lid.

11. Tooth Cleanser

Ingredients:

- 15 drops of Bergamot essential oil

- 10 drops of clove essential oil

- 20 drops of lemon essential oil

- 3 ounces of orris root, powdered

- 1 lb of arrow root, powdered

- 1 ounce of myrrh, finely powdered

- dash of sage, finely powdered

Directions:

In a mixing bowl combine your dry ingredients. Blend them well. Add in the oils and mix them into the mixture. Mix until thoroughly blended. Store in dark glass container with airtight lid.

12. Clove-Lemon Tooth Cleanser

Ingredients:

- 15 drops of Bergamot essential oil

- 10 drops of clove essential oil

- 25 drops of lemon essential oil

- 3 ounces of orris root, powdered

- 1 lb of arrow root, powdered

- 1 ounce of myrrh, finely powdered

- dash of sage

Directions:

In a mixing bowl combine your dry ingredients. Blend them well. Add in the oils and mix them into the mixture. Mix until thoroughly blended. Store in dark glass container with airtight lid.

13. Pamela's Toothpaste

Ingredients:

- 2 drops of peppermint essential oil
- 5 drops of lemon essential oil
- 1/4 of a teaspoon of hydrogen peroxide
- 1 teaspoon of baking soda

Directions:

In a mixing bowl combine your dry ingredients. Blend them well. Add in the oils and mix them into the mixture. Mix until thoroughly blended. Store in dark glass container with airtight lid.

14. Eucalyptus Toothpaste

Ingredients:

- 1 teaspoon of Stevia

- 25 drops of Eucalyptus essential oil

- 8 tablespoons of coconut oil

- 7 tablespoons of baking soda

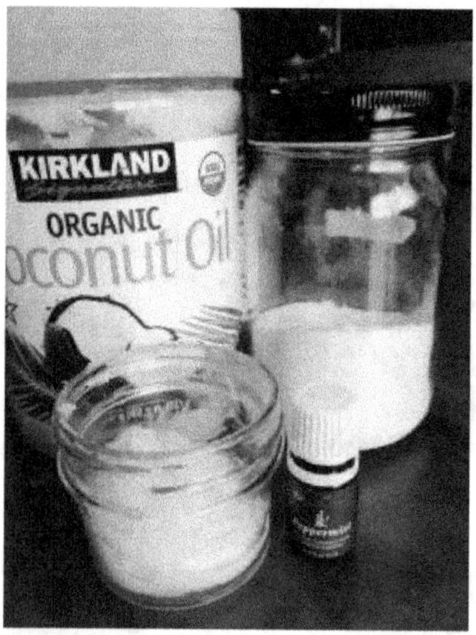

Directions:

In a mixing bowl combine your dry ingredients. Blend them well. Add in the oils and mix them into the mixture. Mix until thoroughly blended. Store in dark glass container with airtight lid.

15. *Lemon Peppermint Toothpaste*

Ingredients:

- 4 tablespoons of coconut oil

- 15 drops of peppermint essential oil

- 8 drops of lemon essential oil

- 1/2 a teaspoon of sea salt, fine

- 3 tablespoons of water

- 4 tablespoons of Bentonite clay

Directions:

In a bowl mix your clay, salt and coconut oil. Add in water a teaspoon at a time as you continue to mix and blend. Use the back of a spoon to "cream" the mixture. Once you have a paste formed add in oil and mix again. Transfer to an opaque container with airtight lid.

17. *Basic Homemade Toothpaste*

Ingredients:

- 1/4 of a teaspoon of hydrogen peroxide

- 1 teaspoon of old fashioned tooth powder

- 5 drops of peppermint essential oil

Directions:

Blend your ingredients well then store them in an opaque container with an airtight lid.

18. Tooth Powder

Ingredients:

- 2 teaspoons of sea salt, fine

- 1/4 cup of baking soda

- 2 tablespoons of dried orange or lemon rind

- 5 drops of lemon essential oil

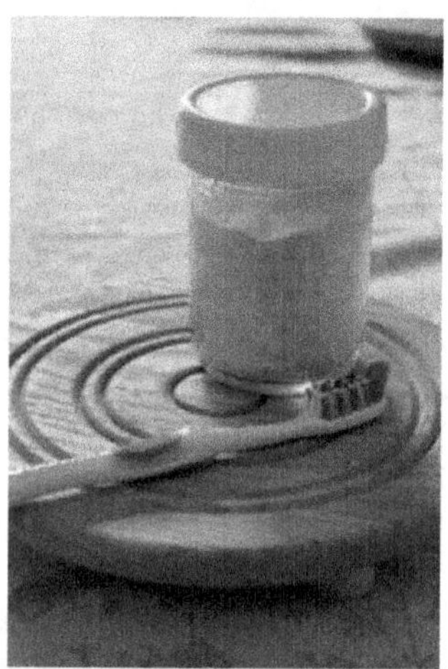

Directions:

Place the rinds inside of your food processor, process them until they become a powder. Add in the salt and baking soda and process for a few more seconds. Add in the lemon essential oil and blend again. Store mix in an airtight container.

19. *All Natural Toothpaste*

Ingredients:

- 1 teaspoon of sage, ground

- 1/4 of a cup of water

- 1/4 of a cup of orris root, powdered

- 1/4 of a cup of arrowroot

- 10 drops of cinnamon essential oil

- 10 drops of clove essential oil

Directions:

Place all of your dry ingredients into your mixing bowl. Slowly add in the water as you mix and blend your ingredients. Stir mix until you form a paste. Transfer the paste into a dark glass jar with airtight lid.

20. Cinnamon Eucalyptus Toothpaste

Ingredients:

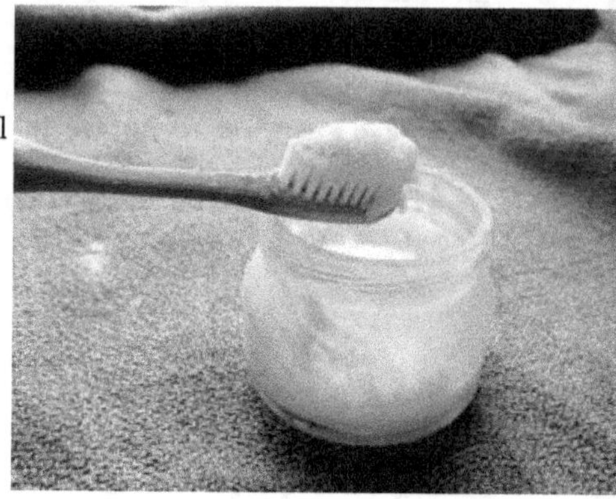

- 15 drops of cinnamon essential oil

- 15 drops of Eucalyptus essential oil

- 1/4 cup of orris root, powdered

- 1/4 cup of water

- 1/4 cup of arrowroot, powdered

- dash of sage

Directions:

Mix your dry ingredients in mixing bowl and slowly add in the water. Then add in the oils and blend until a paste is formed. Store the paste in opaque container with an airtight lid.

Chapter 2. Collection of Homemade Mouthwash Recipes

21. Spearmint Mouthwash

Ingredients:

- 2 ounces of vodka

- 7 ounces of water

- 4 teaspoons of liquid glycerin

- 15 drops of spearmint essential oil

- 1 teaspoon of aloe vera gel

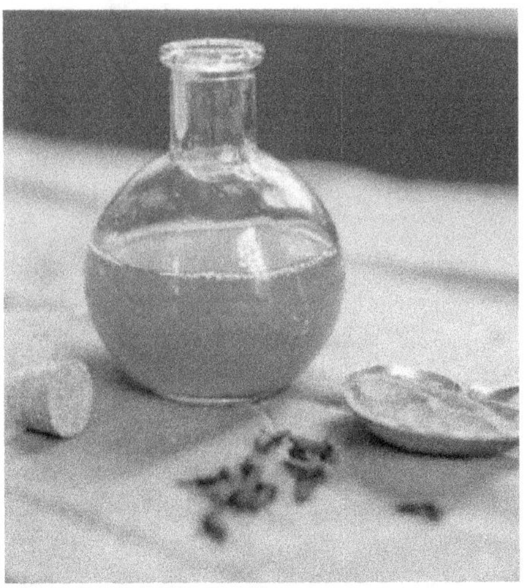

Directions:

In a pan add your vodka and water, placing pan over medium heat to bring to a boil. Add in the glycerin and aloe vera and remove the pan from heat. Allow mixture to cool a bit then add in your oil and mix. Transfer mixture to a bottle and seal with cap. Shake well before each use.

22. *Mint Mouthwash*

Ingredients:

- 2 teaspoons of baking soda

- 20 drops of peppermint essential oil

- 1 tablespoon of witch hazel

- 1/2 a cup of distilled water

- 1 cup of aloe vera juice

Directions:

In a bottle mix all of your ingredients by shaking bottle. Store the bottle in a cool dark place, shelf life is 2 weeks.

23. *Tea Tree Mouthwash*

Ingredients:

- 6 drops of Stevia, liquid

- 5 drops of tea tree essential oil

- 4 drops of peppermint essential oil

- 1 teaspoon of baking soda

- 8 ounces of distilled water

- 1 tablespoon of witch hazel

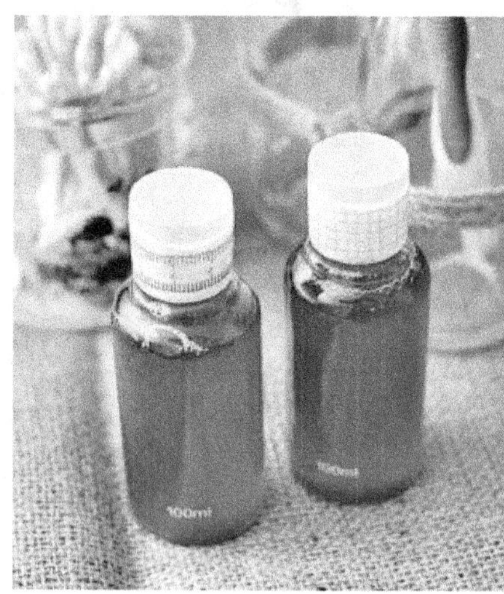

Directions:

Place all of your ingredients into a bottle with airtight lid. Shake well before each use.

24. *Lemon & Tea Tree Mouthwash*

Ingredients:

- 20 drops of lemon essential oil

- 20 drops of tea tree essential oil

- 1 cup of distilled water

- 1 teaspoon of witch hazel

Directions:

Place all of your ingredients into a bottle with airtight lid. Shake well before each use.

25. *Herbal Mouthwash*

Ingredients:

- 1 ounce of rosemary, fresh, chopped

- 1 ounce of Oregon grape root

- 1/2 an ounce of whole cloves

- 2 cups of boiling water.

Directions:

In pan add the water and bring to a boil over medium heat. Add in the other ingredients and allow the mix to steep overnight after removing from heat. In the morning pour ingredients through a cheesecloth into an opaque jar. Store in the fridge, seal with airtight lid. The shelf life for this mouth wash is 1 week.

26. *Hydrogen Peroxide Mouthwash*

Ingredients:

- 5 drops of peppermint essential oil

- 1 cup of distilled water

- 1/4 of a teaspoon of hydrogen peroxide

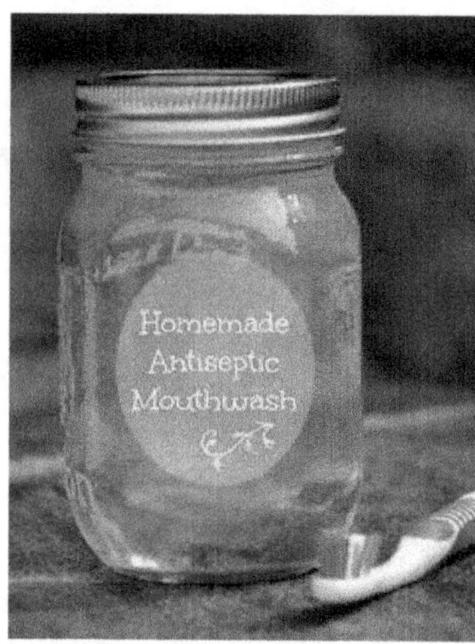

Directions:

Add your ingredients to a bottle with secure lid. Shake well before each use.

27. *Apple Cider Mouthwash*

Ingredients:

- 1 cup of distilled water

- 2 tablespoons of apple cider vinegar

- 10 drops of peppermint essential oil

Directions:

Place all of the ingredients into a bottle with secure lid. Shake well before each use.

28. *Basic Homemade Mouthwash*

Ingredients:

- 1 cup of distilled water

- 1 teaspoon of baking soda

- 4 drops of peppermint essential oil

- 1 teaspoon of witch hazel

Directions:

Add all of your ingredients into a bottle with secure lid. Shake well before each use.

29. Mint & Rosemary Mouthwash

Ingredients:

- 2 1/2 cups of distilled water

- 1 teaspoon of tincture myrrh

- 1 teaspoon of anise seeds

- 1 teaspoon of rosemary leaves

- 1 teaspoon of mint leaves, fresh

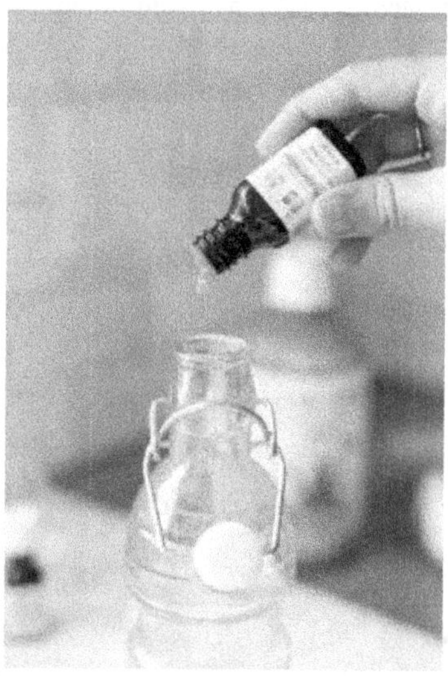

Directions:

Place water in a pan and heat over medium heat bringing to a boil. Add in your herbs and seeds. Allow the mix to infuse for at least 20 minutes. Allow mix to sit overnight. In the morning pour mix through cheesecloth and strain into container that has an airtight lid.

30. Lemon & Ginger Mouthwash

Ingredients:

- 20 drops of lemon essential oil

- 1/2 teaspoon of ginger, powder

- 2 cups of distilled water

- 1 teaspoon of calcium magnesium powder

- 1 tablespoon of witch hazel

Directions:

Mix all of your ingredients in a bottle with a secure lid. Shake well before each use.

31. Basil & Coriander Mouthwash

Ingredients:

- 20 drops of basil essential oil

- 1 teaspoon of coriander, powdered

- 1 tablespoon of hydrogen peroxide

- 2 1/2 cups of distilled water

- 1 teaspoon of Stevia

Directions:

Add all of your ingredients into a bottle with a secure lid. Shake before each use.

32. *Mandarin Mouthwash*

Ingredients:

- 20 drops of Mandarin essential oil

- 5 drops of lemon essential oil

- 1 teaspoon of baking soda

- 2 cups of distilled water

- 1 teaspoon of calcium magnesium powder

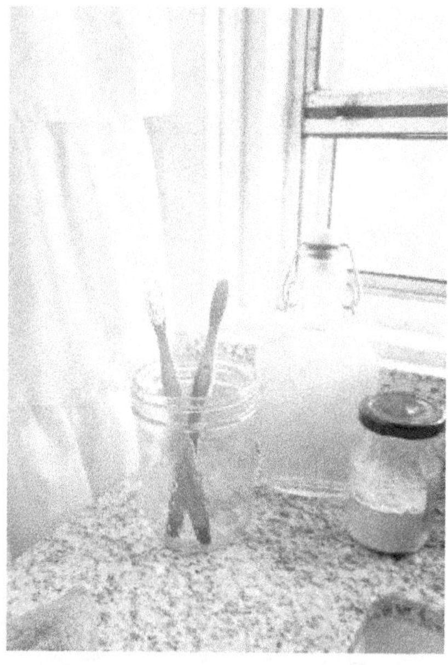

Directions:

Add all of your ingredients into a bottle with a secure lid. Shake before each use.

33. *Anise & Fennel Mouthwash*

Ingredients:

- two cups of boiling water

- 1 teaspoon of anise seeds

- 1 teaspoon of fennel

- 1 tablespoon of witch hazel

- 10 drops of peppermint essential oil

Directions:

First bring your pot of water to a boil add in the fennel and anise seeds and allow mix to infuse for at least 20 minutes. Remove from heat and allow to cool down add in the witch hazel, peppermint essential oil. Store in bottle with secure lid. Shake well before each use.

34. *Whole Cloves & Myrrh Mouthwash*

Ingredients:

- 2 1/2 cups of boiled water

- 1 ounce of myrrh, fine powdered

- 1 ounce of whole cloves

- 1 teaspoon of calcium magnesium powder

- 3 tablespoons of raw honey

- 10 drops of spearmint essential oil

Directions:

In a pot bring the water to a boil over medium heat. Add in the whole cloves and myrrh and mix. Add in the honey and calcium powder and stir in well. Remove from heat and allow to cool adding in the spearmint essential oil. Strain through cheesecloth and store mix in bottle with secure lid. Shake before each use.

35. *Spearmint & Cardamom Mouthwash*

Ingredients:

- 10 drops of cardamom essential oil

- 5 drops of spearmint essential oil

- 4 tablespoons of raw honey

- 1 teaspoon of hydrogen peroxide

- 2 cups of boiling water

- 10 drops of lemon essential oil

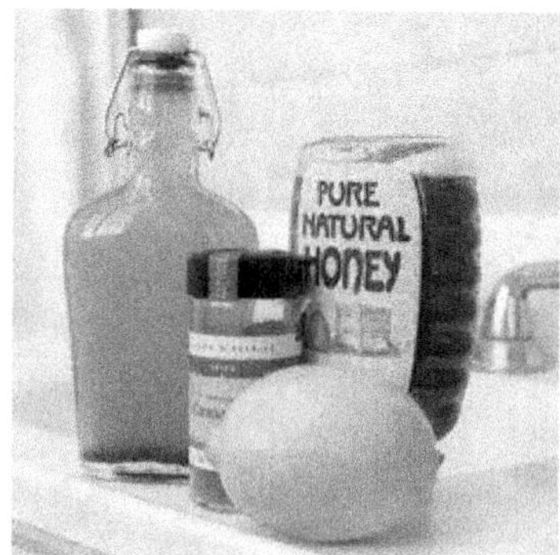

Directions:

Boil your water in pan over medium heat. Add in the honey and mix well. Remove from heat allow to cool down and then add in remaining ingredients. Store mixture in bottle with secure lid. Shake before each use.

36. Peppermint & Patchouli Mouthwash

Ingredients:

- 10 drops of Patchouli essential oil

- 8 drops of Peppermint essential oil

- 2 1/2 cups of distilled water

- 1 tablespoon of witch hazel

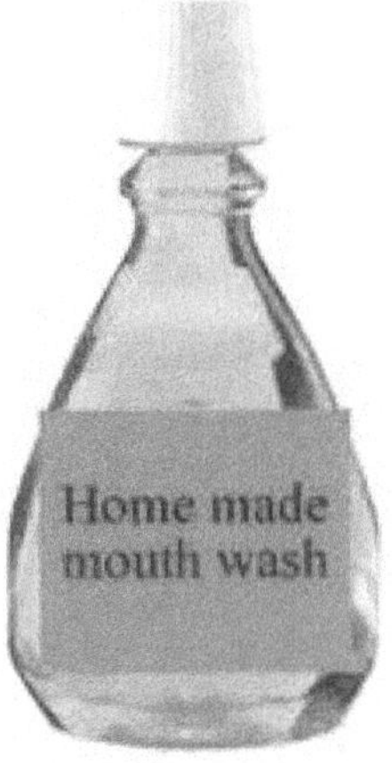

Directions:

Add all of your ingredients into a bottle with a secure lid. Shake before each use.

37. *Orange & Cardamom Mouthwash*

Ingredients:

- 2 1/2 cups of distilled water

- 1 teaspoon of hydrogen peroxide

- 20 drops of orange essential oil

- 15 drops of cardamom essential oil

- 1 teaspoon of apple cider vinegar

Directions:

Add all of your ingredients into a bottle with a secure lid. Shake before each use.

38. *Citrus Mouthwash*

Ingredients:

- 10 drops of mandarin essential oils

- 10 drops of lemon essential oils

- 5 drops of orange essential oils

- 1 tablespoon of witch hazel

- 2 1/2 cups of distilled water

Directions:

Add all of your ingredients into a bottle with a secure lid. Shake before each use.

39. *Peppermint Mouthwash*

Ingredients:

- half a teaspoon of ginger, powdered

- 20 drops of peppermint essential oil

- 2 1/2 cups of distilled water

- 1 teaspoon of apple cider vinegar

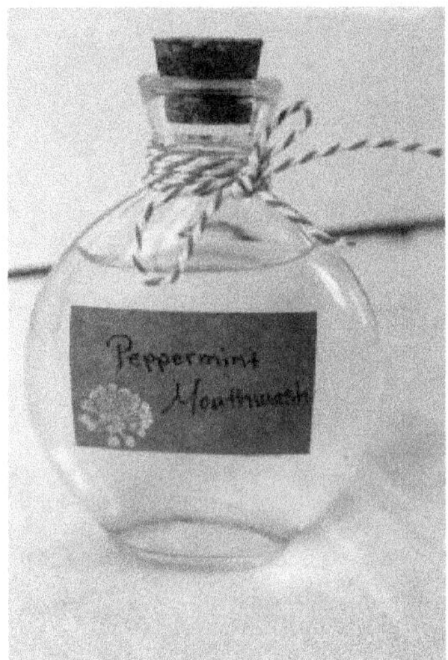

Directions:

Add all of your ingredients into a bottle with a secure lid. Shake before each use.

40. Oregano & Lemon Mouthwash

Ingredients:

- 20 drops of lemon essential oil

- 15 drops of Oregano essential oil

- 1 tablespoon of witch hazel

- 2 cups of distilled water

- 5 drops of peppermint essential oil

Directions:

Add all of your ingredients into a bottle with a secure lid. Shake before each use.

41. SPF Anti-Cold Lip Balm

Ingredients:

- 2 tablespoons of coconut oil

- 1 pastille of beeswax

- two teaspoons of cocoa butter

- 1 1/2 teaspoons of Red raspberry seed oil

- 40 drops of Eucalyptus essential oil

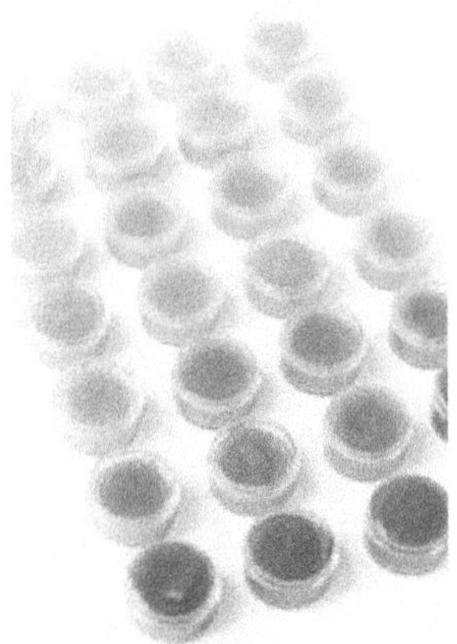

Directions:

Mix your ingredients together and blend them well. You should store your lip balm in a small tin or balm container. The raspberry seed oil is very high in SPF ranging between 30 to 50. This will offer you a very protective lip balm for all seasons.

42. *Homemade Lemon Balm Infused Oil*

Ingredients:

- 3/4 jar full of lemon balm leaves, dried, crumbled
- fill jar 3/4 full of olive oil

Directions:

Stir the contents of the jar then cap the container. Allow the jar to sit in the dark for a period between 4 to 6 weeks.

43. *Anti-Cold Lemon Lip Balm*

Ingredients:

- 4 tablespoons of lemon balm infused oil
- 1/2 a tablespoon of Tamanu oil
- 1 tablespoon of coconut oil
- 1/2 a tablespoon of castor oil
- 2 tablespoons of beeswax
- 1 tablespoon of Shea butter
- 10 drops of tea tree essential oil
- 20 drops of peppermint essential oil
- 3 drops of clove bud essential oil

Directions:

Mix all of your above ingredients you will end up with about 7 1/2 ounces of lip balm. Place your oils, beeswax and Shea butter inside of a heat proof container. Place heat proof container into a pan with some water. Immerse the container into water.

Heat the pan over medium heat, so that your ingredients will melt. Stir the contents remove from pan. Add in your essential oils and stir well. Add mix to small mason jars, or tiny tins, but do not place lids on them yet. Once the lip balm has had a chance to settle into containers then you can put the lids on them. Do not leave your lip balm exposed to light. Using this lemon lip balm will help to get rid of cold sores.

44. *Peppermint Lemon Anti-Cold Lip Balm*

Ingredients:

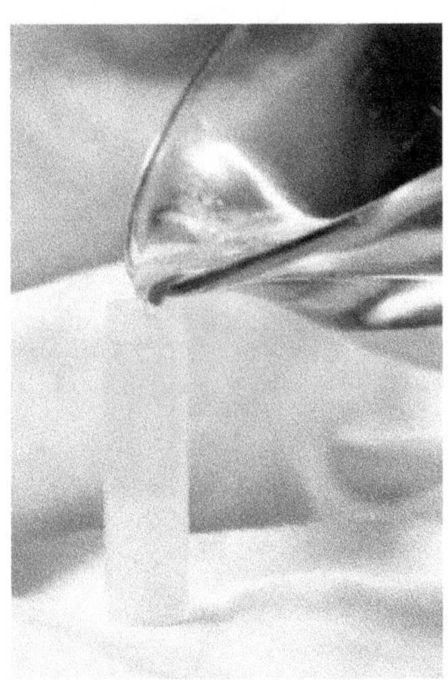

- 20 drops of peppermint essential oil

- 15 drops of lemon essential oil

- 2 tablespoons of beeswax

- 3 tablespoons of Shea butter

- 5 drops of Eucalyptus essential oil

Directions:

In a pan melt your Shea butter and beeswax over low heat. Remove from heat allow to cool down a bit and then add in other ingredients and mix well. Store in lip balm tins, allow to cool and harden by leaving the lid off tins until the balm has firmed. Keep balm in a cool dark place.

45. Mandarin & Jojoba Lip Balm

Ingredients:

- 20 drops of mandarin essential oils
- 1 tablespoon of jojoba oil
- 3 tablespoons of Shea butter
- 2 tablespoons of beeswax
- 1 tablespoon of glycerin

Directions:

In a pan over medium heat melt your beeswax, Shea butter and Jojoba oil. Stir well. Remove from heat and add in your mandarin essential oil and glycerin. Blend ingredients well. Add to lip balm tins, leaving lids off until the balm has had a chance to harden up. Store in a dark cool place.

46. Aloe Vera Lip Balm

Ingredients:

- 1 tablespoon of aloe vera gel

- 3 tablespoons of Shea butter

- 2 tablespoons of beeswax

- 20 drops of Eucalyptus essential oil

- 1 tablespoon of glycerin

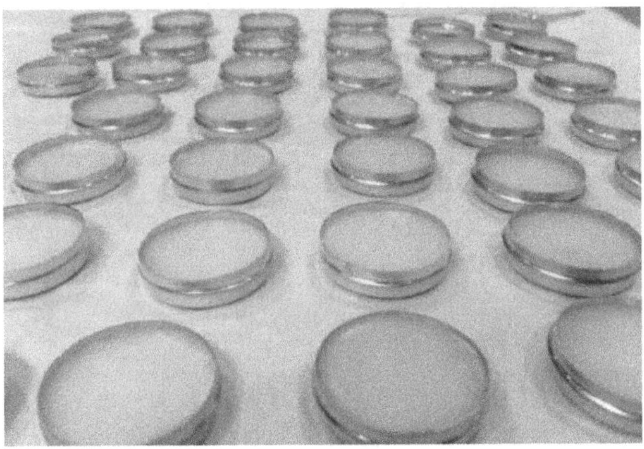

Directions:

In a pan over medium heat melt your Shea butter, beeswax, once melted remove from heat. Add in remaining ingredients and blend well. Add to lip balm tin leaving lid off to allow lip balm to harden slightly then place on the lid and keep in a dark and cool place.

47. *Cinnamon Lip Balm*

Ingredients:

- 20 drops of cinnamon essential oil

- 1 tablespoon of glycerin

- 4 tablespoons of Jojoba oil

- 3 tablespoons of beeswax

- 3 tablespoons of She butter

Directions:

Heat your Shea butter, and beeswax over medium heat, stirring until melted. Remove from heat once melted. Add in remaining ingredients and blend well. Add to lip balm tin. Keep in cool dark place.

48. *Mango & Tea Tree Lip Balm*

Ingredients:

- 1 tablespoon of mango butter

- two tablespoons of beeswax

- 20 drops of tea tree essential oil

- 1 tablespoon of aloe vera gel

Directions:

Melt your beeswax, and mango butter over medium heat in pan. Once they have melted remove from heat. Stir in the remaining ingredients. Add to lip balm tip and let sit for 30 minutes with the lid off. Place lid onto tin and store in dark cool place.

49. Clove Bud Lip Balm

Ingredients:

- 5 drops of clove bud essential oil

- 1 tablespoon of aloe vera gel

- 1 tablespoon of glycerin

- 2 tablespoons of mango butter

- 3 drops of peppermint essential oil

- 2 tablespoons of beeswax

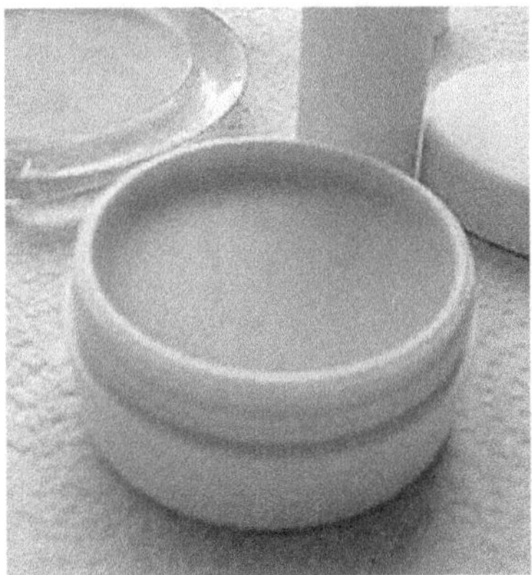

Directions:

In a pan over medium heat melt your beeswax, mango butter, once melted remove from heat. Add in remaining ingredients and blend well. Store in lip balm tin, leave with lid off for about 30 minutes then place lid on and store in cool dark place.

50. Rose Coconut Lip Balm

Ingredients:

- 1/4 cup of beeswax

- 1/8 of a cup of coconut oil

- 1 teaspoon of sweet almond oil

- 1/4 cup of rose petals, fresh or dried

- 1 teaspoon of vanilla extract

Directions:

Measure all of the ingredients into a pan and heat over medium heat, mix well. Pour the mix into lip balm tins and allow to settle by leaving lid off for 30 minutes. You may want to strain the rose petals out, but I like to leave them in it looks nice with them in!

51. Honey & Hemp Lip Balm

Ingredients:

- 2 tablespoons of beeswax

- 2 tablespoons of manuka honey

- 2 teaspoons of hemp oil

- 10 drops of citrus essential oil

- 2 tablespoons of cocoa butter

- 1 tablespoon of Shea butter

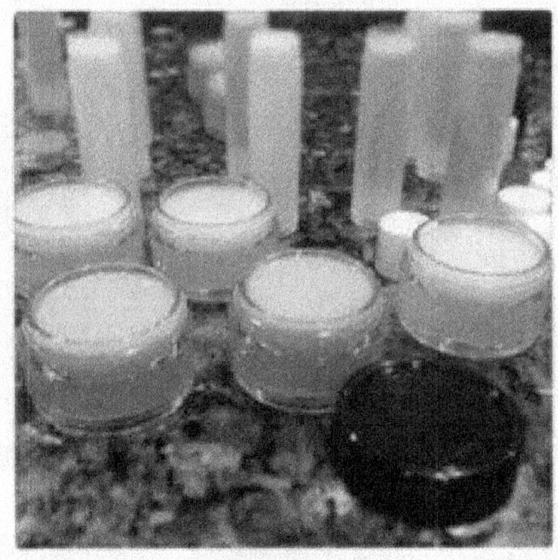

Directions:

Heat in a pan over medium heat your Shea butter, manuka honey, beeswax, cocoa butter. Once they are melted blend well and remove from heat. Add in the remaining ingredients. Store in lip balm tins keep the lid off for about 30 minutes then place lid on and store it in a dark cool place.

52. Strawberry Lip Balm

Ingredients:

- 2 tablespoons of beeswax pellets

- 4 tablespoons of olive oil

- 10 drops of strawberry essential oil

- 2 tablespoons of Mango butter

- 1 tablespoon of glycerin

Directions:

Heat the beeswax, and mango butter until melted over medium heat in a pan. Remove from heat once melted. Add in the remaining ingredients and blend well. Store into lip balm tins keep lids off until balm has hardened. Store in a dark cool place.

53. Vanilla Coconut Lip Balm

Ingredients:

- 1 teaspoon of vanilla extract

- 2 tablespoons of coconut butter

- 1 tablespoon of jojoba oil

- 1 tablespoon of glycerin

- 2 tablespoons of beeswax

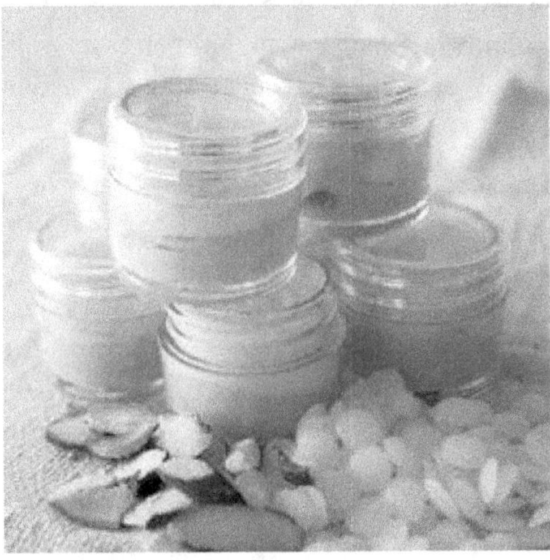

Directions:

Heat the beeswax, and coconut butter in pan over medium heat. Once they have melted remove from heat and add in remaining ingredients and blend well. Store in lip balm tin and keep lid off for half an hour to allow balm to harden up a bit. Store tin in a cool and dark place.

54. *Lemon Vaseline Lip Balm*

Ingredients:

- 20 drops of lemon essential oil

- 3 tablespoons of Vaseline

- 2 teaspoons of beeswax

Directions:

In a microwaveable bowl add in the Vaseline and beeswax. Microwave for 30 second increments until they are melted. Remove from microwave and add in the lemon essential oil and blend well. Store in lip balm tin and keep it in a dark cool place.

55. *Kool-Aid Lip Gloss*

Ingredients:

- 4 tablespoons of petroleum jelly

- 1 package of Kool-Aid powder, flavor of your child's choice

- 1 teaspoon of coconut oil, melted

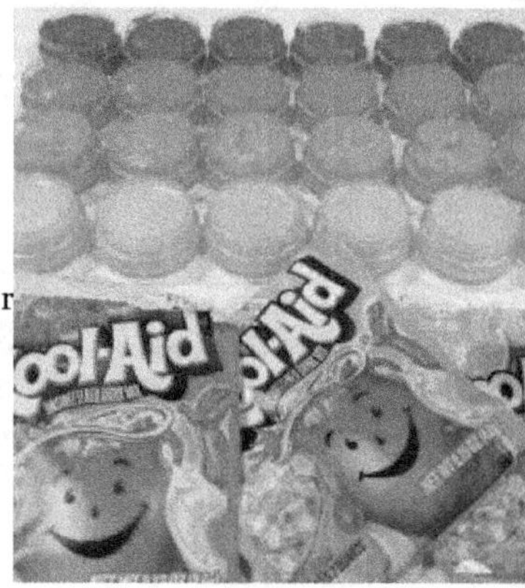

Directions:

In a small bowl bowl mix these ingredients together and make sure to get rid of any lumps. Add the liquid mix to a small container. Do not put the lid on right away and allow it to set for about 20 minutes. Now your child has some great tasting fun lip gloss.

56. *Mango Pineapple Lip Balm*

Ingredients:

- 1 tablespoon of beeswax pastilles

- 1 tablespoon of Shea butter

- 1 tablespoon of coconut oil

- 1 teaspoon of castor oil

- 1/4 of a teaspoon of vitamin E

- 15 drops of mango flavor

- 20 drops of pineapple flavor

- 1/2 a teaspoon of mica powder

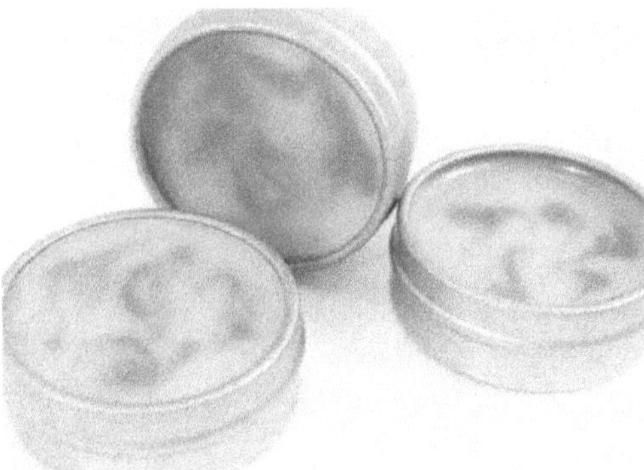

Directions:

In a pan there over medium heat add in the beeswax, Shea butter, and once it is melted remove from heat. Add in all of the other ingredients and blend well. Add into lip balm tin, keep the lid off for about 30 minutes. Place the lid on and keep in cool dark place.

57. *Lime & Coconut Lip Balm*

Ingredients:

- 10 drops of lime flavor

- 15 drops of coconut flavor

- 1 tablespoon of unrefined coconut oil

- 1 tablespoon of beeswax pastille

- 1 teaspoon of avocado oil

- 1/2 a teaspoon of mica powder

- two tablespoons of mango butter

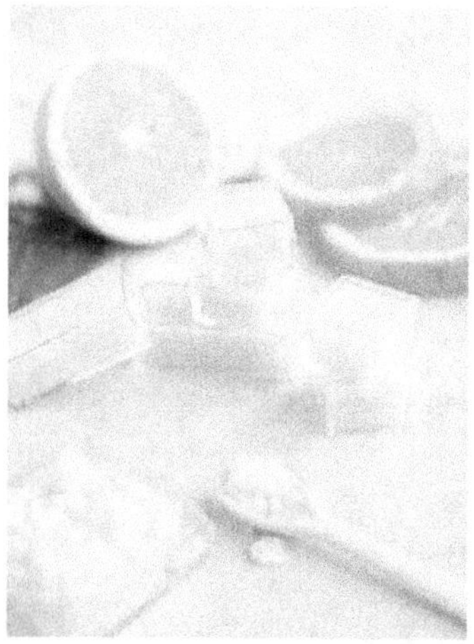

Directions:

Heat in a pan your beeswax, coconut oil, and mango butter over medium heat. Once they are melted remove from heat. Add in the remaining ingredients. Stir and blend well. Add into lip balm tin. Leave lid off for 30 minutes to allow to harden balm up a bit. Add lid then place it in a cook dark place.

58. *Caramel Apple Flavor Lip Balm*

Ingredients:

- 5 drops of caramel flavor

- 25 drops of red apple flavor

- 1 tablespoon of unrefined coconut oil

- 2 tablespoons of Shea butter

- 1/4 of a teaspoon of vitamin E

- 1 teaspoon of rosehip seed oil

- 1 tablespoon of beeswax pastilles

Directions:

Add the Shea butter, beeswax, and coconut oil into pan over low heat. Once they are melted remove from heat. Add in the remaining ingredients. Store balm in lip balm tin, leave lid off for 30 minutes. Place lid on and store it in a cool dark place.

59. Strawberries & Cream Lip Balm

Ingredients:

- Three drops of vanilla flavor

- 25 drops of strawberry flavor

- 1 tablespoon of beeswax pastilles

- 1 tablespoon of mango butter

- 1 teaspoon of castor oil

- 1 teaspoon of jojoba oil

Directions:

In a pan heat the beeswax and mango butter until they are melted. Remove from heat and add in the other remaining ingredients. Blend them well. Add into lip balm tin, leave lid off for 30 minutes. Store in cook and dark place.

60. Chocolate Covered Cherries Lip Balm

Ingredients:

- 5 drops of milk chocolate flavor

- 20 drops of cherry flavor

- 1 tablespoon of beeswax pastilles

- 1 teaspoon of hemp seed oil

- 2 tablespoons of mango butter

- 1/2 a teaspoon of mica powder

- 1 tablespoon of coconut oil

Directions:

In a pan heat the mango butter and coconut oil until they are melted and mixed together. Remove from heat and add in the remaining ingredients. Add mix to lip balm tin, leaving lid off for 30 minutes. Place lid on and store lip balm in a cool and dark place.

Conclusion

I hope that you and your loved ones will enjoy using this collection of natural homemade oral care products. They are easy and cheap to make, will come in handy when you are trying to cut down on costs.

You will be amazed at the kind of savings that you can gain from making more of your own homemade herbal products. They are also much healthier to use than other products that are filled with many chemicals and additives that are out on the market. Feel good when you use your homemade oral care products with the knowledge that you know exactly what went into them!

Thanks again for supporting my work by downloading this book. I appreciate it greatly, I would love to read a review of it by you on Amazon. Take care and happy making your own homemade oral care products!

FREE Bonus Reminder

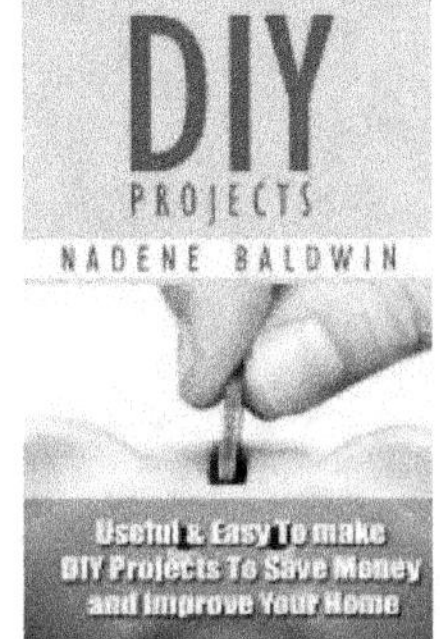

If you have not grabbed it yet, please go ahead and download your special bonus report *"DIY Projects. 13 Useful & Easy To Make DIY Projects To Save Money & Improve Your Home!"*
Simply Click the Button Below

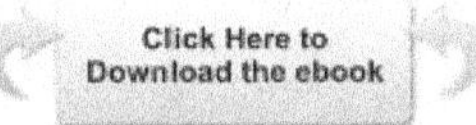

OR **Go to This Page**
http://diyhomecraft.com/free

BONUS #2: More Free & Discounted Books or Products

Do you want to receive more Free/Discounted Books or Products?
We have a mailing list where we send out our new Books or Products when they go free or with a discount on Amazon. Click on the link below to sign up for Free & Discount Book & Product Promotions.
=> Sign Up for Free & Discount Book & Product Promotions <=

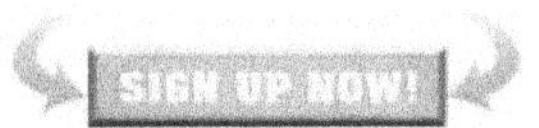

OR Go to this URL
http://zbit.ly/1WBb1Ek